HCG Diet

A Beginner's Overview and Unbiased Review for Women

copyright © 2024 Stephanie Hinderock

All rights reserved No part of this book may be reproduced, or stored in a retrieval system, or transmitted in any form or by any means, electronic, mechanical, photocopying, recording, or otherwise, without express written permission of the publisher.

Disclaimer

By reading this disclaimer, you are accepting the terms of the disclaimer in full. If you disagree with this disclaimer, please do not read the guide.

All of the content within this guide is provided for informational and educational purposes only, and should not be accepted as independent medical or other professional advice. The author is not a doctor, physician, nurse, mental health provider, or registered nutritionist/dietician. Therefore, using and reading this guide does not establish any form of a physician-patient relationship.

Always consult with a physician or another qualified health provider with any issues or questions you might have regarding any sort of medical condition. Do not ever disregard any qualified professional medical advice or delay seeking that advice because of anything you have read in this guide. The information in this guide is not intended to be any sort of medical advice and should not be used in lieu of any medical advice by a licensed and qualified medical professional.

The information in this guide has been compiled from a variety of known sources. However, the author cannot attest to or guarantee the accuracy of each source and thus should not be held liable for any errors or omissions.

You acknowledge that the publisher of this guide will not be held liable for any loss or damage of any kind incurred as a result of this guide or the reliance on any information provided within this guide. You acknowledge and agree that you assume all risk and responsibility for any action you undertake in response to the information in this guide.

Using this guide does not guarantee any particular result (e.g., weight loss or a cure). By reading this guide, you acknowledge that there are no guarantees to any specific outcome or results you can expect.

All product names, diet plans, or names used in this guide are for identification purposes only and are the property of their respective owners. The use of these names does not imply endorsement. All other trademarks cited herein are the property of their respective owners.

Where applicable, this guide is not intended to be a substitute for the original work of this diet plan and is, at most, a supplement to the original work for this diet plan and never a direct substitute. This guide is a personal expression of the facts of that diet plan.

Where applicable, persons shown in the cover images are stock photography models and the publisher has obtained the rights to use the images through license agreements with third-party stock image companies.

Table of Contents

Introduction	7
Background Overview of the HCG Diet	9
What is the HCG Diet?	9
The Invention of the HCG Diet	10
Criticism	11
Potential Side Effects	12
The Structure and Functioning	13
HCG Structure	13
How Does HCG Work?	13
What You Can Eat and What You Can't?	14
Improvement in Body Composition	15
How can you implement the HCG Diet?	16
HCG Diet for Women	18
Diet Analysis	21
Necessary Conditions	21
Pros/Benefits of the HCG Diet	22
Cons of the HCG Diet	23
Usage Instructions	26
When Should the HCG Diet be Used?	26
Resources and Meal Plan	26
Modifications	28
Conclusion	29
Sample Recipes	32
Chicken Apple Wraps	33
Roasted Steak and Onions	34
Whitefish Taco Wraps	35
Oven Roasted Asparagus	36
Roast Tomato Slices	37
FAQ and Summary	38
References and Helpful Links	41

Introduction

Do you want to lose weight quickly without exercise and while still enjoying your favorite foods? If yes, read this concise and professional review of the HCG Diet and follow the prescribed diet plan to get your desired results in a short time.

Data released by the National Health and Nutrition Examination Survey showed the prevalence of severe obesity was 11.5% among U.S women in 2017-2018 (Hales, Carroll, Fryar, & Ogden, 2018). Obesity results in serious health problems among adults including end-stage renal disease, respiratory issues, and coronary heart disease.

Besides, pregnant overweight women face several pregnancy complications like gestational diabetes mellitus (GDM), hypertension, congenital defects, fertility issues, and preeclampsia.

However, you can get rid of obesity and lose weight quickly by following the HCG diet plan, which is claimed to reduce up to 0.5-1 kg of weight per day. The process is highly efficient, safe, and secure and causes fast weight reduction among pregnant women without causing any hunger or weakness.

HCG refers to human chorionic gonadotropin, which is a hormone pregnant women release in large quantities during the early stages. Often used by doctors and gynecologists to test pregnancy, HCG can also treat fertility issues and was proposed as a weight-loss tool in 1954 by Albert Simeons (Palsdottir, 2018).

The HCG diet combines severe calorie restriction (500 calories/day) with the HCG hormone injections (Zeratsky, 2019). You can achieve dramatic weight loss by using HCG products in various forms including pellets, drops, and sprays.

In this HCG diet guide, you will discover:

- What is HCG and who presented the idea of the HCG diet as a weight-loss mechanism
- How effective the HCG diet is to treat obesity
- What are the potential risks or side effects of using the HCG diet
- What researchers, nutritionists, dietitians, and doctors say about the efficiency and reliability of the HCG diet
- Some legal obligations of the HCG diet in the United States
- Final recommendation on whether to use the HCG diet or not

Background Overview of the HCG Diet

What is the HCG Diet?

The HCG is an abbreviation of human chorionic gonadotropin, a protein-based hormone produced by women during the early stages of pregnancy, which occurs from the end of the first week to the beginning of the second trimester

HCG plays a key role in the production of progesterone and estrogen, two very important hormones that boost the development of the embryo and fetus. Hormones are chemicals that regulate the body's crucial processes and influence how organs function. In simple terms, progesterone and estrogen help you conceive and continue to maintain a pregnancy. Deficiency of these hormones can result in infertility or an increased risk of miscarriage.

There are two main components of the HCG diet: An ultra-low-calorie diet and HCG hormone injections. Several randomized trials focusing on the HCG diet revealed the low-calorie diet has a primary contribution to any weight loss among pregnant women.

The HCG dieters have to take a maximum of 500 calories/day for two consecutive months. For this purpose, they can use homeopathic medicines like pellets, drops, or sprays. Besides, you are not allowed to eat much as the HCG diet allows you to have only lunch and dinner. Every meal will comprise one bread, one protein, one fruit, and one vegetable each.

The Invention of the HCG Diet

The HCG was proposed as a weight-loss tool by a British endocrinologist named Dr. Albert T. Simeons in 1954. His research showed the HCG regimen burns extra body fat stored in the hips, stomach, and thighs (Zeratsky, 2019). Besides, Simeons also observed that the HCG dieters do not feel hungry or suffer from any kind of nutrition problems.

Simeons documented his research findings in a book titled Pounds and Inches, which discussed in detail some of the causes of obesity and useful weight-reduction techniques (Simeons, 2010). Later, Simeons combined an ultra-low-calorie diet with daily HCG injections to treat obesity among pregnant women. The combination was named the HCG diet and was aimed at losing adipose tissue without loss of lean tissue.

Based on the findings of Dr. Simeons, the idea of the HCG diet originated, which is an effective and fast weight-reduction plan that allows patients to lose 0.5-1 kg weight per day (Robb-Nicholson, 2010). The HCG diet boosts metabolism and helps women quickly reduce excessive body fat without feeling hungry.

Criticism

Nevertheless, the efficiency of HCG was questioned in several studies conducted in the last quarter of the twentieth century. The Food and Drug Administration received several complaints about the side effects of the HCG diet.

Consequently, the FDA asked Simeons Management Corp. in 1976 to include a disclaimer on their advertisements that stated there was no substantial evidence that weight reduction treatments including the HCG injections reduce weight, redistribute fat, or decrease hunger.

Nevertheless, calorie-restrictive diets were found to be helpful in rapid weight reduction due to caloric restriction.

Moreover, a study conducted by Stein et al. (1976) called HCG less effective than dietary restriction to treat obesity and lose weight. Similarly, a meta-analysis published in 1995 found no scientific evidence supporting the role of HCG in fat redistribution, weight loss, and hunger control (Lijesen, Theeuwen, Assendelft, & Van, 1995).

In 2016, the American Medical Association declared HCG inappropriate as a weight-loss technique based on the findings presented in the 1995 metal analysis (AMA, 2016).

Potential Side Effects

According to certified Dietitian Katherine Zeratsky, extremely low-calorie diets like HCG are risky and may result in a deficiency of vitamins and minerals, irregular heartbeat, an imbalance of electrolytes, and gallstone formation (Zeratsky, 2019).

Other side effects associated with the HCG diet include irritability, gynecomastia, edema, fatigue, depression, and restlessness. In most severe cases, the diet causes thromboembolism and forms blood clots in veins that increase the possibility of a heart attack.

The Structure and Functioning

HCG Structure

The HCG is a glycoprotein having a molecular mass of 36.7 kDa and composed of 237 amino acids (Canfield, O'Connor, Birken, Krichevsky, & Wilcox, 1987). Being a heterodimer, it has two subunits called α (alpha) and β (beta), both of which create a small hydrophobic core. The α (alpha) subunit contains 92 amino acids, while the β (beta) subunit is made up of 145 amino acids. Most of the outer amino acids in HCG are hydrophilic.

How Does HCG Work?

The HCG plays a key role in the maintenance of the corpus luteum by interacting with the LHCG receptor of the ovary. With this process, the hormone progesterone is secreted by the corpus luteum that helps doctors and gynecologists recognize pregnancy at the early stages (Kayisli, Selam, Guzeloglu-Kayisli, Demir, & Arici, 2003). Progesterone also enables the uterus to sustain the growing fetus by providing it with a thick lining of capillaries and blood vessels.

In terms of weight loss, the HCG diet boosts metabolism and burns or redistributes fat. As a result, you can treat obesity and lose weight without feeling hungry. HCG also suppresses hunger pangs by communicating with the hypothalamus (a part of the brain that regulates appetite) and sending signals to release stored fat to provide energy. Thus, the body is able to burn off excess fat without feeling deprived of food.

The HCG also safeguards the fetus during the first trimester by repelling the mother's immune cells. Some researchers also believe the HCG also contributes to the development of local maternal immune tolerance. The hormone also activates apoptosis and participates in cellular differentiation/proliferation.

However, excessive levels of HCG can cause Hyperemesis gravidarum or morning sickness in pregnant women (Askling, Erlandsson, Kaijser, Akre, & Ekbom, 1999).

What You Can Eat and What You Can't?

Since the HCG diet involves a low-calorie diet for rapid weight-loss, you are not allowed to eat much. In the HCG diet plan, you will have only lunch and dinner, each meal comprising one bread, one protein, one fruit, and one vegetable ("HCG," 2019).

Foods Allowed:

- Lean proteins such as chicken, fish, shrimp, and beef (no visible fat)
- Non-starchy vegetables like spinach, lettuce, cucumbers, and tomatoes
- Fruits such as apples, oranges, strawberries, and grapefruit
- Selection of low-carbohydrate bread or grissini (breadsticks)

Foods not allowed:

- High-fat meats like bacon, sausage, and ribs
- Starchy vegetables such as potatoes and corn
- Fruits with high sugar content like bananas, grapes, and mangoes
- Any type of added sugars or sweeteners (honey, agave nectar, etc.)
- High-carbohydrate breads or foods made with white flour

Additionally, you can use sugar substitutes, tea, coffee, and one tablespoon of milk per day. Water is a key ingredient of the HCG diet, hence drink as much water as you want.

Improvement in Body Composition

Low-calorie diets like the HCG not only reduce body weight, but also decrease muscle mass (Chaston, Dixon, & O'Brien,

2007). Besides, the body tries to conserve energy by burning fewer calories because it thinks it is starving.

On the other hand, the supporters of the HCG diet reject the concept that this diet affects body muscles in addition to fat loss. Instead, they claim consuming the HCG diet boosts metabolism and results in an anabolic state by elevating other hormones.

Nevertheless, all these claims are hypothetical with no scientific evidence to prove their validity. Hence, if you are on a low-calorie diet, you can burn your body fat without losing muscles by eating high-protein foods, weightlifting, and doing a 30-minute workout daily.

How can you implement the HCG Diet?

The doctors have divided the HCG diet plan into three phases, which are given below:

Loading Phase

During the first phase, the body undergoes preparation for caloric restriction by storing normal fat cells, thereby enhancing the process of fat burning. To initiate this phase, the patient begins taking HCG (Human Chorionic Gonadotropin) and consumes a high-calorie diet consisting of foods rich in fats for a duration of two days, accompanied by daily HCG injections. This approach not only helps in reducing hunger but also helps in minimizing the initial adverse effects that may arise due to low-calorie intake.

Weight Loss Phase

In this second phase, the patient continues consuming HCG supplements and follows a strict 500 calories/day diet for a period of 3-6 weeks. This phase is designed to promote rapid weight loss. If you are looking to achieve your weight loss goals quickly, it is recommended to repeat these phases several times until you observe a substantial improvement in your weight and overall health.

Maintenance Phase

Once the weight loss phase is completed, the patient transitions into the maintenance phase. During this phase, the intake of HCG is gradually stopped, and the patient gradually increases their food consumption over a period of 3 weeks. However, it is important to note that the use of sugar and starch is strictly prohibited during this phase. The maintenance phase aims to stabilize the weight loss achieved during the previous phase and establish healthy eating habits for long-term weight management.

HCG Diet for Women

There are plenty of dieting options for women to lose weight and improve body texture including the Apple Cider Vinegar Diet, the Tapeworm Diet, Cookie Diet, and the Air Diet. However, none of these diets match the efficiency and competence of the HCG diet.

Invented by a British endocrinologist Dr. Albert T. Simeons in 1954, the HCG diet is an eight-week diet plan that combines a low 500-calorie diet with HCG injections for rapid weight loss. According to clinical dietitian Bethany Doerfler, HCG is an FDA-approved hormone often used by gynecologists to treat infertility (Kassel, 2017).

Women who are on the HCG diet are injected 125 units of human chorionic gonadotropin (HCG) hormone six days a week consistently for 3 to 6 weeks. It is an expensive treatment as each shot of the HCG injections costs up to $250 to $600 and boosts metabolism along with a fast breakdown of body fat.

Additionally, the weight-loss process speeds up by cutting calories as the patients are allowed to intake a maximum of

500 calories a day. You can eat two meals per day comprising one vegetable, 3.5 ounces of meat, and one bread slice. Besides, high-cholesterol foods, oils, and exercise is strictly prohibited, and you can take only one tablespoon of milk every 24 hours.

Moreover, women need to sacrifice a lot while on the HCG diet as they cannot use any cosmetics or body lotions other than lipstick, even after special permission.

Nevertheless, despite severe criticism and long-held outrage by the scientific community, the HCG diet plan helps women lose weight. Renowned bariatric physician Dr. Spencer Nadolsky does not consider the HCG diet an effective program to treat obesity and calls starvation or a low-calorie diet the primary factors behind weight loss (Nadolsky, 2014).

He argues that the HCG injections do not boost the pound-shedding process. Instead, by eating extremely low-diet fat, your body starts losing muscles rather than fat, which results in a slowed metabolic rate. Temporarily, you feel you are getting rid of obesity and losing weight but once you stop taking the low-calorie diet, everything is back.

Another flaw in the weight-reduction plan of the HCG diet for women is the lack of exercise, which is essential to losing fat. The reason behind that a low-calorie diet is insufficient to fulfill your daily energy needs.

Let alone exercise, I do not have sufficient energy to get up early in the morning and have a walk. Hence, no exercise means more muscle loss which is extremely dangerous, particularly for pregnant women.

Considering the homeopathic or over-the-counter (OTC) nature of HCG products, the Food and Drug Administration has not approved the HCG diet. Even doctors, dietitians, and nutritionists are not allowed to prescribe HCG for weight loss and it is illegal to inject HCG hormones other than fertility treatment.

From this discussion, it can be concluded that the HCG diet is an expensive, unsustainable, and extremely dangerous weight-loss practice. There is no other way to treat obesity quickly than doing exercise regularly and eating a balanced diet to fulfill your energy requirements.

Even if you intend to try the HCG diet, you must consult your gynecologist and get the necessary information about its risks and benefits to avoid any irreparable loss.

Diet Analysis

Necessary Conditions

The HCG diet works by limiting the calorie intake and injecting HCG hormones to lose weight quickly. The energy contents in daily food consumption are measured in calories. However, several risks are also associated with the HCG diet, particularly if you're a pregnant woman.

The following conditions must be fulfilled while you are on the HCG diet.

- You must take HCG injections or drops daily;
- Drink as much water as you can;
- Seek medical advice from a qualified physician;
- Consume low-calorie foods like vegetables, foods, and bread;
- Avoid consuming high-cholesterol foods, oils, sugar, and alcohol
- Always use fresh fruits and vegetables; and
- Weight your food before consumption.

Pros/Benefits of the HCG Diet

Rapid Weight Loss

The HCG diet is known for its ability to trigger rapid weight loss in the initial stages, with patients following a strict 500-calorie-per-day regimen. However, it is important to note that health experts argue there is no scientific evidence supporting the role of HCG hormone injections in fat reduction or redistribution. Instead, the dramatic weight loss observed is primarily attributed to the significantly restricted calorie intake.

Natural and Versatile

One of the unique aspects of the HCG diet is that it utilizes a hormone that is 100% natural and extracted from humans. Apart from its use in weight loss, HCG is also employed in the treatment of infertility. This makes the HCG diet a viable option for women, as it does not pose any harmful implications. It is worth mentioning, though, that some temporary side effects may manifest at the beginning stages.

Hormonal Balance and Libido Enhancement

Maintaining a balanced hormonal profile is crucial for both mental and physical well-being. As an important hormone, HCG aids in regulating hormonal levels, thereby reducing the risk of dysfunction. Additionally, HCG stimulates endocrine activity and has been reported to improve libido levels.

Result-Oriented and Structured Plan

The HCG diet plan offers a well-structured, performance-oriented blueprint that aims to produce tangible results. From its well-delineated three phases to the daily calorie targets and prescribed units of hormonal injections, this diet provides clear instructions for women to follow and adhere to. This organized approach contributes to the ease of implementation and compliance with the diet plan.

Appetite Suppression

A common struggle faced by many individuals striving to lose weight is controlling their appetite and resisting their favorite foods. The HCG hormone, however, has been found to effectively reduce appetite and diminish the cravings for more food. By curbing hunger pangs, the HCG diet aids in achieving significant weight loss.

Cons of the HCG Diet

Potential Risks and Importance of Professional Guidance

The HCG diet can be potentially risky, and its effectiveness may not be realized unless undertaken under the guidance of a qualified dietitian or physician. Failing to consult with a professional may result in undesired outcomes such as weight gain or the loss of muscle mass, which can negatively impact physical health.

Lack of Adequate Nutrition

Due to the low-calorie nature of the HCG diet, certain high-cholesterol foods such as dairy and grains, which are important sources of essential proteins and fats necessary for physical and mental growth, are restricted. The avoidance of these foods may lead to a deficiency in nutrition, particularly among pregnant women.

Legal Restrictions

It is important to note that the Food and Drug Administration (FDA) has prohibited the consumption of HCG in the United States, except for its approved use in treating fertility issues. Consequently, it is illegal for doctors to prescribe the HCG diet as a weight loss aid.

Potential Side Effects and Health Concerns

The use of HCG can potentially cause various side effects in the body, including headaches, depression, swelling, and fatigue. Moreover, excessive intake of HCG hormone may result in the development of ovarian hyper-stimulation syndrome and even premature puberty in young boys.

Safety Considerations and Cardiac Health

The HCG diet entails keeping the body in a state of prolonged calorie restriction for several weeks, which can lead to a deficiency in protein. In response, the body may start extracting proteins from the heart, potentially causing hazardous contractions known as ventricular tachycardia. Additionally, the use of HCG supplements may contribute to the growth of excess breast tissue in men.

While the HCG diet offers potential benefits in terms of weight loss and hormonal balance, it is important to consider the associated risks and consult with healthcare professionals before embarking on this diet plan.

Usage Instructions

When Should the HCG Diet be Used?

The HCG diet plan allows a maximum of 500 calories per day in two meals. Although there is no definite timing for these two meals, most of the dietitians equally divide these calories between lunch and dinner. This means you will be taking 250 calories at lunch and 250 calories at dinner.

Similarly, you can take tea or coffee in your breakfast, but without any sugar. Instead, you can use stevia or saccharin for sweetening purposes (Garone, 2020). One tablespoon of milk can also be added to your coffee or tea at breakfast time.

Resources and Meal Plan

There are no specific recipes required by the HCG diet. You can achieve your desired results as long as you follow the guidelines about daily calorie intake and eat compliant foods.

However, you can also find customized meal plans and useful tips on different websites to follow the 500-calorie-per-day target. Based on data collected from different resources, given below is a weekly meal plan for the HCG diet (Hannan, 2020).

Days	Breakfast	Lunch	Dinner
Monday	Water, tea, coffee	Chicken orange, steamed asparagus, breadstick	Tilapia, strawberry, salsa, spinach
Tuesday	Water, tea, coffee	Melba toast, super bef chili	Tilapia, strawberry, salsa, lettuce salad
Wednesday	Water, tea, coffee	Chinese orange, beef stir-fry	Chicken cacciatore, breadstick
Thursday	Water, tea, coffee	Chicken cacciatore, breadstick	Chinese orange, beef stir-fry
Friday	Water, tea, coffee	Grilled chicken breast, tangy apple slaw	Broiled lemon, garlic shrimp, Melba toast, lettuce salad
Saturday	Water, tea, coffee	Broiled lemon, garlic shrimp, spinach salad, Melba toast, lettuce salad	Tangy apple slaw, bodacious burger
Sunday	Water, tea, coffee	Breadstick, super beef chili	Lettuce salad, fresh basil, chicken with orange

Modifications

Most of the dietitians recommend the 500-calorie plan of the HCG diet. However, Dr. Richard Lipman presented an alternative 800-calorie plan almost similar to the one presented by Dr. Simeons.

Although Dr. Lipman's plan also eliminated sugar, carbohydrates, and high-cholesterol foods, it offered a broader and more diversified variety of food options (Garone, 2020). Besides, the 800-calorie plan is more satisfying, but most people claim it leads to less dramatic weight loss.

Conclusion

HCG is a hormone produced in women during the early stages of pregnancy. It helps gynecologists confirm pregnancy and is often used to treat infertility.

The HCG diet is a rapid weight-loss mechanism that combines an ultra-low calorie diet with HCG hormone injections. The idea of using HCG hormones to treat obesity was first presented by a British endocrinologist Dr. Albert T. Simeons in 1954. Since then, the HCG diet has been consumed by many individuals, particularly women, to burn their body fat and reduce weight without doing exercise.

However, most of the research and health experts consider the HCG diet an inefficient, unsafe, and dangerous weight-loss method. Several studies focusing on the outcomes of the HCG diet found no scientific evidence to suggest the diet can help in rapid weight reduction without any side effects.

Instead, doctors recommend other sensible and safe weight-loss methods like exercising and eating a balanced diet. The HCG diet is a potentially dangerous practice to shed pounds.

Considering the side effects and serious health concerns arising from the use of the HCG diet, the Food and Drug Administration has not approved this plan as an aid for weight loss. It is even illegal for doctors in the United States to use HCG hormone for any treatment other than to cure fertility issues.

According to Leonard (2018), individuals who are on an HCG diet may suffer from various side effects like fluid buildup in body tissues, blood clotting, mood changes, and enlarged breasts in males.

Other reported side effects of the HCG diet include fatigue, restlessness, depression, irritability, edema, gynecomastia, thromboembolism, and lack of energy. Besides, the ultra-low-calorie diet can cause low mood, malnutrition, gallstones, irregular heartbeat, electrolyte imbalance, vitamin deficiency, diabetes, muscle loss, kidney disease, and increased risk of gallstones.

Taking only 500 calories per day can cause a severe deficiency of proteins and vitamins in the body since a low-calorie diet is insufficient to fulfill daily energy needs. Besides, a study conducted by Parikh, Thomas, Raguckas, and Shi (2015) concluded the HCG diet is not suitable for losing weight as it neither alleviates hunger nor redistributes body fat.

The legality of the HCG diet is also questionable in different countries. For instance, the sale of over-the-counter (OTC) products containing HCG has been banned in the United States by the Federal Trade Commission (FTC) and the Food and Drug Administration (FDA).

Based on the researchers' findings and the doctor's recommendations, it can be concluded that HCG is a fad diet with no substantial evidence supporting its role in treating obesity. You may observe little improvement in the start as you intake a low-calorie diet, but severe calorie restriction can attack your muscles.

Hence, it is recommended that instead of trying the HCG diet as a weight-loss mechanism, you should exercise regularly and take a balanced diet.

If you are interested in reading more information about the usefulness of the HCG diet for women, read the following resources.

1. HCG 2.0 by Dr. Zach LaBoube
2. The HCG Diet Fact and Fiction by Adele Frizzell
3. New 800 Calorie HCG Diet by Richard L. Lipman

Sample Recipes

Chicken Apple Wraps

Ingredients:

- 100 g diced chicken
- 1 small apple, diced
- 2 tablespoons lemon juice
- 1/8 teaspoon cardamom
- Stevia
- 1/8 teaspoon cinnamon
- Salt
- Pepper
- Smoked paprika

Instructions:

1. Cook 100 g diced chicken with a dash of salt, pepper, and smoked paprika until fully cooked.
2. Add the diced apple to the cooked chicken.
3. Sprinkle 2 tablespoons of lemon juice over the mixture.
4. Add 1/8 teaspoon of cinnamon and 1/8 teaspoon of cardamom for a delightful flavor.
5. Sprinkle a pinch of stevia for a touch of sweetness.

Roasted Steak and Onions

Ingredients:

- 100 g flank steak (no fat)
- 1 onion, sliced
- Water

Instructions:

1. Heat a medium-sized skillet and add 100 g flank steak.
2. Brown the steak on both sides until nicely seared.
3. Place the steak in a preheated oven and broil until cooked to your desired level of doneness.
4. Add one small sliced onion to the pan.
5. Add a splash of water to deglaze the pan.
6. Sauté the onions until they reach your desired level of caramelization.

Whitefish Taco Wraps

Ingredients:

- 100 g whitefish
- ¼ cup of water
- 1 clove crushed garlic
- ½ teaspoon chili powder
- Iceberg lettuce leaves
- Salt and black pepper
- ¼ teaspoon ground cumin

Instructions:

1. Evenly coat the whitefish with crushed garlic, chili powder, salt, black pepper, and ground cumin.
2. Bake the seasoned fish in a preheated oven at 350°F until the fluids run clear.
3. Remove the fish from the baking dish and lightly break it up using a fork.
4. Spoon the flaked fish into crisp iceberg lettuce leaves for a refreshing taco experience.

Oven Roasted Asparagus

Ingredients:

- 1 bunch of asparagus
- 1 clove minced garlic
- 1 tablespoon lemon juice
- 3 tablespoons water
- 1 teaspoon salt
- Black pepper

Instructions:

1. Preheat the oven to 425°F.
2. Dip the asparagus in a mixture of water and lemon juice for a burst of tangy flavor.
3. Sprinkle the asparagus with minced garlic, salt, and black pepper.
4. Arrange the seasoned asparagus on a baking sheet in a single layer.
5. Bake the asparagus for 12-15 minutes until it reaches the desired tenderness.

Roast Tomato Slices

Ingredients:

- 1 tomato
- 1 sprig rosemary
- Chopped garlic
- Salt
- 1 clove crushed garlic

Instructions:

1. Cut the tomato into thin slices.
2. Spread the tomato slices on a parchment paper-lined cookie sheet.
3. Sprinkle the tomato slices with chopped rosemary, garlic salt, and a touch of salt for enhanced flavor.
4. Sandwich the crushed garlic between the tomato slices.
5. Roast the tomato sandwich at 200°F for approximately 6 hours until it reaches a rich, roasted texture.

FAQ and Summary

Q1: What is the HCG diet?

A1: The HCG diet is a weight-loss program that combines daily injections of the HCG hormone with a 500 to 800 calorie diet. The diet is based on the theory that HCG helps the body burn fat faster, thus promoting weight loss.

Q2: How does the HCG diet work?

A2: The HCG diet works by encouraging the body to burn stored fat for energy. The diet is low in calories and targeted at rapid weight loss. The HCG hormone injections are believed to curb appetite and maintain muscle mass, despite the low-calorie intake.

Q3: Is the HCG diet safe for women?

A3: It's important to note that the HCG diet restricts calorie intake significantly, which can lead to nutrient deficiencies and other health risks. Therefore, it's crucial to consult with a healthcare professional before starting the HCG diet.

Q4: How long does the HCG diet last?

A4: The HCG diet is typically split into three phases: the Loading phase, which lasts for two days; the Weight Loss phase, which can last anywhere from 3 to 6 weeks; and the Maintenance phase, which continues for 3 weeks after stopping the HCG injections.

Q5: What can I eat on the HCG diet?

A5: The HCG diet primarily includes lean proteins, vegetables, and fruits. However, the intake is limited to 500 to 800 calories a day, and all meals are devoid of fats, sugars, and processed foods.

Q6: Are there any side effects of the HCG diet?

A6: Some potential side effects of the HCG diet can include fatigue, irritability, restlessness, and in some cases, depression. Moreover, the low-calorie intake can lead to nutrient deficiencies, leading to hair loss and muscle weakness.

Q7: Does the HCG diet work for everyone?

A7: The effectiveness of the HCG diet can vary from person to person. It's essential to consult with a healthcare practitioner to determine if the HCG diet is the right choice for your individual health needs and weight loss goals.

Q8: Can I exercise while on the HCG diet?

A8: Light exercise, such as walking or gentle yoga, is typically allowed on the HCG diet. However, strenuous exercise is generally discouraged due to the low-calorie intake.

Q9: Can men follow the HCG diet?

A9: Yes, men can also follow the HCG diet. However, they should consult with a healthcare professional before starting, as HCG is a hormone that naturally occurs in pregnant women, and its effects on men are less well-studied.

Q10: Can I drink alcohol on the HCG diet?

A10: Alcohol is generally not allowed on the HCG diet due to its high-calorie content and potential to hinder weight loss progress.

In conclusion, while the HCG diet for women promises rapid weight loss, it's essential to remember that it involves drastic changes in diet and hormone intake. Therefore, it should be undertaken with caution and under the supervision of a healthcare professional.

References and Helpful Links

AMA. (2016). Use of HCG in the Treatment of Obesity. American Medical Association.

Askling, J., Erlandsson, G., Kaijser, M., Akre, O., & Ekbom, A. (1999). Sickness in pregnancy and sex of child. Lancet, 2053.

Canfield, R., O'Connor, J., Birken, S., Krichevsky, A., & Wilcox, A. (1987). Development of an assay for a biomarker of pregnancy and early fetal loss. Environmental Health Perspectives, 57–66.

Chaston, T., Dixon, J., & O'Brien, P. (2007). Changes in fat-free mass during significant weight loss: a systematic review. International Journal of Obesity, 743-750.

Garone, S. (2020, November 05). What Is the HCG Diet? Retrieved from https://www.verywellfit.com/the-hcg-diet-4688734

Hales, C. M., Carroll, M. D., Fryar, C. D., & Ogden, C. L. (2018). Prevalence of Obesity and Severe Obesity Among Adults: United States, 2017–2018. National Center for Health Statistics.

Hannan, M. (2020). The Complete HCG Diet Plan. Retrieved from https://www.hcgdietinfo.net/hgc-diet-plan-food-list/

Kassel, G. (2017, December 27). Considering the HCG Diet? Here's What You Need to Know. Retrieved from https://www.womenshealthmag.com/weight-loss/a19977570/hcg-weight-loss/

Kayisli, U., Selam, B., Guzeloglu-Kayisli, O., Demir, R., & Arici, A. (2003). Human chorionic gonadotropin contributes to maternal immune tolerance and endometrial apoptosis by regulating the Fas-Fas ligand system. Journal of Immunology, 2305–2313.

Lijesen, G., Theeuwen, I., Assendelft, W., & Van, D. W. (1995). The effect of human chorionic gonadotropin (HCG) in the treatment of obesity by means of the Simeons therapy: a criteria-based meta-analysis. British Journal of Clinical Pharmacology, 237–43.

Nadolsky, S. (2014, May 01). The Fat Loss Workout I Prescribe to my Patients. Retrieved from http://drspencer.com/the-fat-loss-workout-i-prescribe-to-my-patients/

Palsdottir, H. (2018, October 15). What Is the HCG Diet, and Does It Work? Retrieved from https://www.healthline.com/nutrition/hcg-diet-101

Robb-Nicholson, C. (2010). By the way, doctor: What do you know about the HCG diet? Retrieved from https://www.health.harvard.edu/newsletter_article/what-do-you-know-about-the-hcg-diet

Simeons, A. T. (2010). Pounds & Inches: A New Approach To Obesity. Popular Publishing.

Zeratsky, K. (2019). Has the HCG diet been shown to be safe and effective? Retrieved from https://www.mayoclinic.org/healthy-lifestyle/weight-loss/expert-answers/hcg-diet/faq-20058164

www.ingramcontent.com/pod-product-compliance
Lightning Source LLC
LaVergne TN
LVHW051926060526
838201LV00062B/4708